The
B.I.B.L.E. W.A.Y
to Health

Prescriptions from the
Great Physician

Bro. Dr. Franco Taylor

For permission requests, write to the author at the address below.
brofranco.rs@gmail.com
Memphis, Tennessee

This book was edited, formatted, designed, and published by:
UNIQUE PUBLISHING HOUSE, LLC
P.O. Box 750792, Memphis, TN 38175
www.uniquehouse.org

ISBN-13: 979-8-9895627-8-7

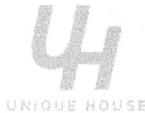

UH
UNIQUE HOUSE

The
B.I.B.L.E. W.A.Y
to Health

Prescriptions from the
Great Physician

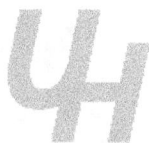

UNIQUE HOUSE

Dedication

This book is dedicated to two sets of people: All of those who have followed Dr. Franco's God-inspired *The B.I.B.L.E.W.A.Y. to Health: Prescriptions from the Great Physician* and, afterward, were blessed to have gained their optimum health; and all of those who will gain their optimum health, after reading this book for the first time, adhering to the pathway to health suggested in *The B.I.B.L.E.W.A.Y. to Health: Prescriptions from the Great Physician.*

Disclaimer Message to the Reader

The purpose of this book is to enlighten and educate. The information presented in this book is not intended as a cure for any ailment or disease. Neither is this book intended to offer medical advice. Therefore, feel free to contact the author through email, for further communications about the B.I.B.L.E.W.A.Y to health. The information in this book is not intended to replace medical treatment or advice. For specific health problems, consult your physician for guidance.

Acknowledgments

I thank God for inspiring me to write *The B.I.B.L.E.W.A.Y. to Health: Prescriptions from the Great Physician*, and I am grateful and indebted to all who played a role in the publication of this work, especially my wife, Linda Redmond Taylor, Ana Washington - my apprentice, and Dr. Candace Jones and the Unique Publishing House, LLC.

I thank my mentor and friend, Bro. Mamon Wilson, Gospel/Medical Missionary/Evangelist, for allowing me to gain practical experience serving as, first, an apprentice, and later, as an instructor, at his sanatorium, the Centurion Bible School of Health in Cypress Inn, Tennessee. I also thank the hundreds of pastors, private business persons, family reunion chair persons and entrepreneurs who hosted "health revivals" and private group presentations to help spread the "gospel" of the B.I.B.LE.W.A.Y. to health's principles to thousands of people in the United States and abroad. Through such gatherings, God's plan for health and wealth continues to be furthered.

Lastly, I thank my nine children, host of family members, and scores of friends who allowed me to gain more knowledge and experience as they adopted the Biblical prescriptions for health, outlined in *The B.I.B.L.E.W.A.Y. to Health: Prescriptions from the Great Physician.* These prescriptions are based on deliberate, exhaustive research and God's direction.

Table of Contents

Foreword

Claudette Jones Shepherd, M.D.

Health is a state of complete physical, mental, and social well-being, and not merely the absence of disease and infirmity. World Health Organization

The medical community has sought to improve the health of individuals and the community at-large in two ways, by implementing programs that increase awareness of disease, and by striving to educate populations about adherence to prescribed therapies. These have often included medications with harsh side effects for which, then, additional medication was needed. Even though modern technology has allowed for continued improvement in medications and earlier diagnosis of many ailments, significant improvements have not been made in overall quality and quantity of life.

The *Healthy People Initiative*, sponsored by the U. S. Department of Health and Human Services, was developed more than four decades ago to address health needs. It brought awareness among health professionals that matters could be simplified. Dr. Louis W. Sullivan, in his foreword to the *Healthy People 2000*, stated that, "We could be terribl[y] remiss if we did not seize the opportunity presented by health promotion and disease prevention to dramatically cut healthcare costs, to prevent the premature onset of disease and disability, and to help all Americans achieve healthier, more productive lives." The initiative of *Healthy People 2010* continues to strive to increase the length and quality of lifestyles, and to eliminate disparities in health status.

Thousands of years ago, under Divine inspiration, holy men of God documented His counsel to His people, designed to promote longevity. When adhered to, it had the effect of preserving the people for service. As a result, it is not surprising that among the 10 Leading Health Indicators described in *Healthy People 2010*, seven are covered in *The B.I.B.L.E.W.A.Y. to Health: Prescriptions from the Great Physician.* Close attention to biblical principles of health ensures not only longer life, as science is now concluding, but also quality of life – years that can be enjoyed to the fullest.

Dr. Franco Taylor has dedicated his life to developing an understanding of these principles and seeking creative means to share with others the remedies and knowledge he has discovered to work. As you read *this book*, you will find a simple yet proven plan that has worked for thousands of years. It transcends all cultures and socioeconomic groups. It is inexpensive to implement and requires only a teachable spirit.

To ward off disease or recover health, men, as a rule, find it easier to depend on the healers than to attempt the more difficult task of living wisely. **Hippocrates**

Preface

There is a great deal of truth in the saying that man becomes what he eats. **Gandhi**

I must have wisdom to be a faithful guardian of my body. **White, 1931**

And said, If thou wilt diligently hearken to the voice of the Lord thy God, and wilt do that which is right in his sight, and wilt give ear to his commandments, and keep all his statutes, I will put none of these diseases upon thee, which I have brought upon the Egyptians: for I am the Lord that healeth thee. **Exodus 15:26**

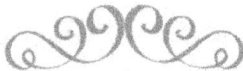

A Righteous Prayer

Brother Dr. Franco Taylor

Our most gracious heavenly Father, the only God who spoke all things into existence except man, we thank You for this ability to use the medium of the written Word to reach many who might have otherwise fallen into disease and death. God, secondly, we thank You for forming man of the dust of the ground, breathing into his nostrils the Breath of Life, and allowing him to become a living soul – that was one example of Your initial love for mankind. With the creation of man, You put into his heart an unmatchable ability to be able to understand Your good and perfect will. Thirdly, we thank You for having the foresight to give us the Holy Bible for us to use as a guidepost to health, wealth and spiritual happiness on earth, and as an ultimate Manual on how to live so that heaven may be our final destination.

Father, help us reach those who may be failing in health, or those who only need to be boosted up to a higher quality of good health. May we write, through You, simple and edifying words that will leave no doubt about what Your desire is for man's lease of his body, for him to present it to You, holy and acceptable - not someday in the future, but right now. May each person who reads this book, be like the woman at the well – urgently desiring to tell all about how they, too, may achieve better health. So, bless us then, we pray to get some tidbits of wisdom that we can use to bring a higher quality of life to ourselves, our families, and those with whom we come into contact. Thank You in advance for the victory over sin in our lives and over the disease in our bodies. In Jesus Christ's name we pray. Amen.

Just as no lecture, counseling session, or sermon should begin without a brief prayer to the One who gave mankind; 1) the *breath* he uses to talk, 2) the *mind* he uses to reason, 3) the *brainpower* he uses to internalize knowledge, 4) the *Spirit* he uses to discern Godly interpretation and experience heavenly revelations, and 5) the *body* that is used as a temple to house that Spirit, so I dared not to begin this book without lifting up thanksgiving and blessings to the One who has kept me throughout 44 years of teaching His natural ways to be well and stay well.

To begin, what comes to mind when the word <u>way</u> is heard? Biblically, that word is used many times, which exemplifies a significance. A search of '<u>way</u>' revealed these Scriptures among many:

Teach me thy way, O Lord, and lead me in a plain path, because of mine enemies. **Psalm 27:11**

Teach me thy way, O Lord; I will walk in thy truth: unite my heart to fear thy name. **Psalm 86:11**

For the commandment is a lamp; and the law is light; and reproofs of instruction are the way of life. **Proverbs 6:23**

Behold, I will do a new thing; now it shall spring forth; shall ye not know it? I will even make a way in the wilderness, and rivers in the desert. **Isaiah 43:19**

More importantly, however, after finding that there are good ways to follow and there are evil ways to follow, there is only one real *way* that counts: Jesus says in John 14:6, "…I am the way, the truth, and the life: no man cometh unto the Father, but by me." Read and heed this carefully: Just as there is only one *way* to God, I am going to boldly, without hesitation or equivocation, state that there is only one *way* to true health. I posit that *way* is the B.I.B.L.E. *W.A.Y.*

Chapter 1

Best Foods and Combinations

> Behold, I have given you every herb bearing seed, which is upon the face of all the earth, and every tree, in the which is the fruit of a tree yielding seed; to you it shall be for meat. **Genesis 1:29**

Grains, fruits, nuts, and vegetables constitute the diet chosen for us by our Creator ... They impart a strength, a power of endurance, and a vigor of intellect by a more complex and stimulating diet. **White, 1951**

Just as Christ was before *Finding Success in Health the B.I.B.L.E. W.A.Y.* was written, the principles outlined as the BIBLEWAY to health existed before there was a U.S. Surgeon General, a National Cancer Institute, or an American Heart Association. The latter ones receive much attention in the world, and many people rely on their advice and dictates. However, as this book is read, everyone will find that it was God who *first* admonished all of the laws of health to which mortal man, *later*, laid a claim. God's Word stands as a testament, and it is time to give tribute to the Holy Bible as the true and authentic authority upon which all other good health books are based. That's right, all lesser lights of health shine because of the One Who gives light.

I am writing to set the record straight: When God said, "For I am the LORD, I change not" (**Malachi 3:6**), He meant it. There is no way that He could have commanded sound laws or practices of health, even as long ago as six thousand years, only to later have those same laws to be decreed of none effect or less importance for the people of today by those who think to be able to change God's laws. One weak line of reasoning is that those laws are outdated because they were for "the Israelites", back then. Were Adam and Eve Israelites, per se? I submit that, just as the Ten Commandments still stand today, noted by prominent pastors who advocate that their parishioners even begin posting them in their homes and offices, the biblical laws of health still stand. Obedience to them means internal order and health. I believe that adherence to them, overall, means life. Disobedience to them means disease and death.

So, the question that will ring throughout this writing will be: *Wilt thou be made whole?* Most times, one's health is in one's own hands. Health is personal, just like choosing to obey the laws on the highway is personal, especially when a person is driving alone. When no one is in the back seat directing the driver's steering wheel and braking for him, the driver either obeys the rules of the road or does not obey them. One thing is sure, a driver's practices will eventually be revealed. Guess what, a person's health practices will eventually be revealed, also. A pure disregard for stop signs, i.e., eating foods that God commands not to eat; yield markers, i.e., refusing to remain within God's will; cattle crossings, i.e., refusing to be temperate; and rest stops, i.e., disregarding His suggestions of systematic resting may all show up later as catastrophic illnesses such as cancer, diabetes, AIDS, colon problems and tumors, whereas, failing to ease over forewarned bumps, i.e., not getting adequate sunshine or refusing to slowly go around curves, i.e., disobediently eating bad combinations of foods, could mean, present, minute inconveniences such as intermittent headaches or being merely overweight that may develop into more serious health challenges later.

The good news, however, is that, with every disease, there is an emergency roadside service station. There, every disease known to man may be fixed, God willing. The only way that it would not be fixed would be that the person did not seek help soon enough. Even then, once the laws of health were totally applied, the body could still make a serious attempt to heal itself. In other words, a renewed level of optimum health could evolve.

Actually, there are eight natural laws upon which true health is based. Following these laws of health, for many, will result in true health and happiness. All one has to do to follow the laws of health, I repeat, is to consult God's Owner's Manual called the Holy Bible. God created human beings and left the instructions for their maintenance so that all of their parts, which by the way, are custom-built, could always be serviced by their Maker. I know this may sound redundant, but repetition is one of the keys to remembering.

God knew that any other instructions would be adulterated and ill-advised and/or even half-truths, since many in the healthcare profession desire to live as upper-class citizens and, therefore, depend on the monies gleaned from sick folks to help them support their lifestyles. Is that why many illnesses are professed to be incurable, but manageable, so that there is always the need for patients to return, continuously, over, and over to the doctor? Anyone who is bothered by God's words through me may go on and say, *"ouch"*. Most times, however, people only become defensive and offended by words when they are directly linked to the words- be it personally or by the knowledge of someone else directly linked to what is said. Now is the appointed time for all guilty practitioners to change their ungodly ways of sacrificing the health of others to gain earthly wealth, if that has been their way of livelihood. God is not pleased because He made man to subdue the earth and to cause the lower animals to be at his command - not to subdue man and cause man to be at his command. All men were created equally. There is nowhere in the Bible where God directs doctors to hold other men under their thumbs by withholding sound advice to them, thereby deliberately making perpetually sick slaves of them.

If, however, physicians are unable to overcome greed, and are unable to realize their mission in life (to assist in the healthful upkeep of the body) God has ordained that every man or woman who is of a sound mind, should study for him or herself. The reality is that no man should allow another man to control him so much that he heeds a mortal man's advice over God's advice. What is wrong with a person when he/she says that the doctor's advice does not make him well or physically stronger, yet, he keeps on following their ill advice? What is the matter with a man and woman when they hear that God desires them to be well and has dictates, actually, simple remedies, that would assist the body in overcoming most illnesses- yet they turn their backs on God's sound advice?

Maybe people who continue to be bound by sickness just have not had an avenue of escape before *The B.I.B.L.E.W.A.Y. to Health: Prescriptions from the Great Physician.* Maybe, without a plain path, many have fallen to disease and death. No more is that reason usable. The simple outline of God's will for man to have health begins close to where the problems begin- with food.

As you have probably gathered, the "**B**" in the acronym *B.I.B.L.E.W.A.Y.* represents "*best food and combinations.*" In order to know what the best foods and combinations of foods are, we must carefully study God's original plan for man's diet.

Immediately after God created the perfect man and woman (Adam and Eve) in His own image, He gave them two commands. First, in Genesis 1:28, He told them 'to be fruitful and multiply as husband and wife, and to replenish the earth with more little perfect beings just like themselves to give Him (God) the honor, praise, and glory'. Secondly, and just as importantly, Genesis 1:29 states that God gave Adam and Eve the best foods to eat in order to keep their perfect bodies clean, strong, and vibrant forever: fruits, nuts, and grains.

Just imagine man in the beginning, tall and majestic, in God's own image, reaching way up into the trees and vines, to pluck the fruits, nuts and grains that God had so graciously planted in the garden for him. As he reached up toward heaven to gather the golden grains, the amber nuts, and luscious fruits, he was saying, "Thank you, God for the free gift of food." In the beginning, man did not have to bend over and work to pick his food; nor did he have to get his fingernails dirty digging on or under the ground for food. On the other hand, the lower animals had to root on, above and beneath the ground to get the vegetables that God commanded them to eat in Genesis 1:30. So, in the Garden of Eden, Adam was commanded to eat only fruits, nuts and grains.

When and why did man get the approval to eat vegetables? For the answer to that question, Genesis. 2:16 and 17 will be examined. Does everyone know the story of how Adam and Eve ate fruit from the one tree that God had forbidden them to eat? Because of their disobedience, sin, sickness and death entered into the world. The ravaging effects of disobedience to God's natural law are *still* being felt. Immediately after sin, and because of sin, God added the food He had dictated for animals to eat, vegetables, to man's diet, and commanded him to work and sweat for his food (**Genesis 3:17-18**). Though this was not in the original, perfect diet given man by his Creator in the beginning, it was still a very good diet. On this diet, Adam, Noah, and Methuselah lived to be over nine hundred years of age.

Of course, this was not as good as living forever and never dying, but it was and is much better than the sixty to seventy years that man lives to be today. However, the question is still on the board: Why did God recommend that man eat vegetables? I posit that vegetables were added to man's diet as a remedial effort to heal his sin–sick body, mind and soul.

One needs only to look at Adam's actions before and after sin to understand this next reasoning. Just before Adam sinned, the Bible states that his body and mind were in perfect condition (**Genesis 1:31**). Further proof of this is in **Genesis 2:19 and 20**, when God gave Adam his first test. God wanted to see if Adam's mind was on one accord with His; so, He gave Adam the responsibility of naming all of the animals that He had made. Adam gave the animals the exact names that God would have given them. Adam passed the test so well that in the very next verses **Genesis 2:21-25**, God rewarded Adam with a wife, Eve. As a side note, when a man's mind is on one accord with God's, he is then capable of loving and caring for a wife physically, mentally, and spiritually, and God can then bring the woman unto the man. It is important to note that, before sin, Adam had a mind that was on one accord with God. Also, God communed openly with Adam and, later, with Eve, after uniting them in marriage (**Harrell, 1991**).

How was Adam's mind after sin? What was the state of his mind after sin? Did Adam have a healthy mind? Immediately after sinning, Adam and Eve heard the voice of the LORD God walking in the garden, and, instead of running *to* meet Him as they usually did, they hid *from* Him (**Genesis 3:8**). After Adam and Eve heard God's "voice", they became full of fear and mistrust. Are these signs of healthy minds or sick minds? These signs usually are instantaneous. For example, when a person sins and decides to tell the first lie, he has to immediately begin weaving "tangled webs' and remembering each lie that is told from that point on. This process becomes tedious for or on the body, to the point of even, possibly, causing high blood pressure and headaches.

In the next verse **Genesis 3:9,** God's "voice" asked Adam "Where art thou?" The answer is simply, "Here I am, Lord"; but, instead Adam answers, "I heard thy voice in the garden, and I was afraid because I was naked; and I hid myself." To picture Adam dodging and unable to look God straight in the face to give a straight answer is a sad sight. God, who is a God of second, third, fourth… chances, tries to get Adam to come straight again and says, *"Who told thee that thou was naked? Hast, thou eaten of the tree whereof I commanded thee that thou shouldest not eat?"* The perfect mind would have answered, " No one told me I was naked. And yes, I have eaten of the tree whereof you commanded me not to eat." But instead, Adam answered *"The woman whom thou gavest to be with me, she gave me of the tree, and I did eat."* So again, Adam dodges God's relevant question, and this time he blames the woman and even God, Himself, for his sinful actions.

Eve, like Adam, cannot give a straight answer to God's *voice's* question, "What is this that thou hast done"? The honest answer would have been along these lines: "I sinned and ate the forbidden fruit, and I persuaded Adam to do the same." Instead, she lays the blame on the serpent (**Genesis 3:13**). I, therefore, posit that fear and mistrust for God, inability to face God's voice and tell Him the truth, shifting the blame and even laying blame on God's "voice", Himself, is proof that after sin, Adam and Eve were physically, mentally, and spiritually sick.

So why did God allow man to eat food that was originally given to the animals (vegetables)? The scriptures tell us that life is in the blood. Good blood flow leads to a good life physically, mentally and spiritually. On the other hand, poor blood flow leads to poor physical, mental, and spiritual life. I, therefore, contend that, after sin, poisons and toxins from wrong eating and stress from disobedience tainted the blood streams of Adam and Eve, thus, adversely affecting their mental clarity. In other words, they had lost their minds. I also contend that God had placed substances in vegetables that acted like medicine, yielding a remedial effect on the tainted bloodstream of man!

"What is he talking about?" is probably the question. One only has to look at the scientific world for further proof. Science has discovered this phenomenon: the molecular structure of human blood and the molecular structure of chlorophyll (the blood of plants) is identical. I repeat, it is identical! The only difference is that Heim or iron is in the center or nucleus of a molecule of blood, and magnesium is in the center or nucleus of a molecule of chlorophyll. The fact that the chlorophyll of plants is identical to blood led me to another discovery. Both the Cancer Institute and Cancer Society have done over twenty-five years of research on the effects of the phytochemicals in certain vegetables on the immune systems of man. The Designer Foods Program yielded astonishing results! The substances in certain cruciferous and other vegetables, (e.g., asparagus, broccoli, turnips, cauliflower, Brussel sprouts, ...) when eaten, block and inhibit the growth of cancer and AIDS cells! The picture becomes quite clear from that bit of information. God gave man vegetables as medicine to heal his sick body and mind. In other words, I believe that God gave Adam and Eve vegetables that contained healing chlorophyll (which was similar to blood) once Adam and Eve sinned. This, in turn, acted as a blood transfusion to heal their weakened states, sin-sick bodies, deranged minds, and tainted blood streams. I'll go one step further to state that this was the beginning of the redemption story: blood sacrifice was necessary to save mankind.

At some point, someone a person knows will be told that he/she needs to have a blood transfusion. That procedure is often given as a last resort to help a person stay alive because of an accident or surgery need, or because of a blood disorder or some other disease. Many are wary of blood transfusions, mostly, because there are possibilities of diseases being transmitted from contaminated bloods. The following statistics may help in making a crucial decision about receiving a transfusion: H.I.V. is transmitted 1 in 1.5 million donations; Hepatitis C occurs 1 in 1.2 million donations, and bacterial contamination occurs in 1 in 100,000 transfusions (**Cleveland Clinic, 2024**).

My mentor, Bro. Mamon Wilson, believes in the revitalization of weak patients who suffer from a low blood count because they are not producing enough hemoglobin. All in all, he suggests that his "iron drink" might be tried to help counter the need for a blood transfusion. His experience has taught that 'if the entire program he suggests is followed for thirty days, a person's red blood count will rise, and the need for a transfusion is often not necessary' (**Wilson & Wilson, 2010**).

One extra tidbit of information is that it costs more to autologously receive a blood transfusion. That is, when a person receives his or her own blood, it's more expensive than receiving it from a random donor. Praise God that His transfusion was all about the saving of lives and the preservation and extension of the health of the human body. Anything that he does or commands is for sustaining, without fear of side effects.

So, fruits, nuts and grains were included in the original, God-given diet. I submit that, if God gave vegetables after sin, as a remedial diet and not the ultimate original diet, then the eating of the flesh of dead animals (which was allowed much later) was never intended as food for man who was created in the image of God. I know that statement will cause a lot of contention. However, there are numerous sources from which raw data has been compiled to confirm that the consumption of blood and fat of animal flesh is against optimum health and natural healing. For example, this is a partial list of animal diseases communicable to man: Tuberculosis, anthrax, foot and mouth disease, Malta fever and abortion disease, milk sickness, swine erysipelas, cox-pox, glanders, rabies, psittacosis and certain parasite diseases, plague, tularemia, infectious jaundice, rat-bite fever, and rocky mountain spotted fever" (**White, 1951; Kloss, 2005**).

This book is not intended to provide an in-depth discussion about the hazards of animal flesh consumption. However, I would be remiss if I did not give the following *food for thought*. God allowed man to continue eating the flesh of animals after the great flood was over and vegetation had been replenished on the earth for one reason. That reason was because man lusted for it (**Deuteronomy 12:15, 20, 21**). Flesh-eating for the purpose of acquiring protein in the diet is a cop out. One does not need to chew on a piece of fried chicken or barbecued ribs in order to "get sufficient amounts of all the proper types of proteins needed by the human body" **(Nedley, 1998).** God knows the needs of His creation. He would rather that his people go back to the original diet. By doing so they would see all sicknesses and diseases slowly disappear from man. One important note to remember: When a person eats a lot of flesh meat, he would do well to eat a raw vegetable salad or raw fruits (for meals that don't include vegetables); this aids in the digestion of the meal (**Kloss, 2005**).

Poor diet along with an inadequate exercise regimen are lifestyle choices that cause most premature deaths every year. Heart and blood vessel disease was the leading affliction that caused death in this country in 1995. Secondly, cancer caused its high share of deaths. "Those facts show that diet has a vital influence on health" (**Nedley, 1998**). This has to be true because, initially, God outlined what foods He desired his human creations to eat. I will repeat that throughout my lifetime - that one fact is most important to grasp.

What are the best combinations of fruits, nuts, grains and vegetables? Vegetables and fruits should not be eaten together at the same meal because they digest at different rates of speed. Fruits digest in from one to one-and one-half hours; vegetables, on the other hand, may take from two to three and even sometimes as many as four hours depending upon factors such as the starch content. When fruits and vegetables are consumed together, fermentation takes place when digested fruit receives excessive gastric juices secreted by the stomach to break down the heavier vegetables. The result is bloating, flatulence, and griping, i.e., sour stomach, pain, and gas passing. No, this was not in God's plan.

Before I end this chapter, I will inform you of the following: God also intended for His people to eat a certain amount of food each day. For instance, He tells everyone in Ezekiel 4: 9–10 how much weight of wheat and barley, beans and lentils, and millet and fitches should be made into bread and eaten each day, i. e., the size of an individual serving. Verse 10 states: "Thy meat, which thou shalt eat should be by weight twenty shekels a day." So, He tells man, who was created in His image, with his perfect body, how much food it will take each day to operate his body properly.

So, in closing, I will suggest one last finding: Fruits should be eaten with a meal that does not include vegetables, e.g., breakfast, and vegetables should be eaten with meals that will not include fruits, e.g., lunch and/or supper.

NOTE: About fruit combinations: acid fruit and alkaline fruit should never be eaten at the same meal. Why? The two opposites, when combined, also cause fermentation and gaseous build-ups in the digestive tract. In other words, sweet fruits, e.g., bananas, figs, and raisins should never be eaten with sour fruits, e.g., oranges, grapefruit, pineapples, and strawberries. Sub-acid fruits, however, i.e., apples, peaches, pears, plums, blueberries, mangoes, and grapes combine well with either the sweet or sour fruits mentioned above.

A minimum of 40 to 50 per cent of every plate of food eaten should be raw. Why? Because there were no stoves or microwave ovens in the Garden of Eden, and neither will there be any stoves or microwave ovens in heaven. God created man to eat his food straight from the trees and vines from which they grew. Cooked food is dead food. Since we are living beings created in the image of God, we should, therefore, eat more of the natural foods containing fiber and living enzymes; these are only found in fresh, raw, uncooked foods, or foods in their natural state.

I realize that I have given a lot of information in this first chapter. After the first reading of the BIBLEWAY, a review would be wise. Contrary to popular beliefs, "meat and milk" do not corner the market on factors that build endurance or strength. Many studies have been conducted that provide scientific evidence about the benefits of the vegetarian diet. It outranks all diets in building/enhancing endurance and strength. One has only to look at the diet of the cheetah, panther, and tiger, and compare it to the diet of the ox, horse and elephant. Overall, the former has speed; the latter has endurance and strength. To be a tiger or an elephant, isn't it good to not have to choose? More on the myths about "meat and milk" later.

Chapter 2

I ntake of Plenty of Water

> *Thou shalt drink also water by measure, the sixth part of an hin: from time to time shalt thou drink.* **Ezekiel 4:11**

Next to oxygen, pure water is the most vital factor to the survival of life. **Bragg & Bragg, 1970**

The second letter of the B.I.B.L.E.W.A.Y. is an "**I**". As aforementioned, That "I" represents "Intake of Plenty of Water". It has been found that water is one of those substances that people will tell me real quickly, "I don't like water"; "I don't like the taste of water"; "I just don't drink water"; "I drink a lot of other types of liquids, e.g., juice and tea"; or, "I drink a lot of Kool-Aid, pops, sodas, fruit waters or whatever that might be available that's sweet, but water is just one of those things that I just can't drink a lot of ". And, oftentimes, when I'm talking to people about water, I ask the question as to why they don't drink it. Most use the following as the bottom-line statement: "I just don't like the taste of it." (More will be discussed about the "taste" of water, later.)

Well, I have this to admonish about that crucial letter "I", which I will state again that it represents "intake of plenty of water". Just as a car's owner's manual dictates the kind and amount of fuel it takes for optimum automobile operation, so it is with God; His manual does the same for the optimum operation of the human body.

In Ezekiel 4:11, God tells everybody how much water should go into these created bodies for optimum performance. It reads thusly: "Thou shalt drink also

24

water by measure, the sixth part of an hin: from time to time shalt thou drink." So, what does that mean in today's terms? If the human body is likened to a car, the car had a designer and a maker. It was Henry Ford. Also, the human body had a Designer and a Creator. It was God. In Ford's owner's manual, people are given instructions on the Ford car's total care, e.g., what octane of fuel or gasoline should go into the gas tank; he tells them what weight and how much oil should go into the crankcase, and how much water should go into the radiator. God does the same with these marvelous machines or bodies that He made for man and woman. In His owner's manual, the Bible, He tells them how much food and how much water should go into it. He also divulges what type of water should go into it. So, water will be the main discussion here.

Again, the scripture reference pertaining to the intake of water is found in Ezekiel 4:11. In the previous chapter, "Best Food and Combinations", it was declared that being well meant being obedient to God's natural laws of health; those words also stand in reference to water:

Exodus 15:26 reads in a paraphrase, thusly: 'If they (the Israelites) will diligently listen to the voice of their God, and do what is right in his sight, and will listen to His commandments and keep all His statutes, He will put none of the diseases upon them that He placed on the Egyptians.' They are being urged to keep God's commandments! How about that? So, since Ezekiel 4:11 begins with the words, "Thou shalt drink... .", it signifies a command, doesn't it? Even though such statements that include the word "shalt" are not in the Ten Commandments, they are commands, nevertheless. So, here, it is seen that God is giving man commands of how much water to drink.

Everyone, please read these next words with a clear and open mind. The following words are also found in the Bible, *God's Owner's Manual*: "Thou shalt drink also water by measure". So, God is saying that man should drink a measured amount of water every day. It goes on to command that "a sixth part of an hin (h-i-n), from time to time shalt thou drink." Now what is a "hin", that a person might get a sixth part of it? Research finds that an "hin", in the Hebrew language, is part of a *bath* of water. It equals approximately a gallon and a half of water, or six quarts. The Bible instructs everyone to drink "one-sixth of a hin."

"So, if the hin is a gallon and a half, or six quarts, and the Bible says to drink it from "time to time", then, is there an exact measurement? Since it is recommended to drink a quart of water at least twice a day (once in the morning and once in the evening), I surmise that everyone should drink one quart of water at least two times a day. Does the reader see where this is leading? One quart is one sixth of six quarts. Six quarts is a gallon and a half, or a hin. Therefore, it would be wise to drink each quart in increments of eight-ounce servings, for optimum water absorption into the body's cells. By the way, the above "hin" summation was revealed to me by God's Holy Spirit because I'm not a mathematician.

Readers, by all means, research my water hypothesis further, and, if it proves to be faulty or in error, I am open for correction. However, let me ask this pertinent question that may shed more light on the issue of drinking water: How many quarts of water do doctors recommend that their patients drink a day? NOTE: Two quarts of water equals eight glasses.

Or better yet, how many glasses of water do doctors and medical professionals tell patients, and have been telling them for the last 30 to 40 years, that they should drink every day? That's right; eight glasses are highly recommended. So, I posit to you that I'm mighty thankful that man has finally caught up to the recommendation of the Great Physician. And, furthermore, I congratulate physicians for finally catching up to where God has been, at least, for over four thousand years. Remember, it was God who commanded man to drink a required amount of water each day. God used His prophet, Ezekiel, to be His mortal mouthpiece to tell His people just how much water to drink in order for their bodies to function healthfully: eight glasses of water, minimum, each day. Now, many people could drink more water than that on a daily basis, and many people should, but the bare minimum for everyone to drink is eight glasses.

Research has shown that adequate water drinking, combined with a healthy lifestyle as described in the BIBLEWAY prescriptions, may actually postpone or prevent many diseases and their complications. Among these illnesses are high blood pressure, heart disease, diabetic complications, and stroke. If a person has chronic or sporadic leg pain, the cure may be found by turning up more glasses of water. Is that simple or what? It has even been found that the more water that smokers drink, the less concentrated are the toxins and poisons that are inhaled from the cigarette smoke.

What about the aged? Would their health improve with more water intake? Some researchers estimate that, if an elderly member of the family is encouraged to drink more water on a daily basis, hospitalizations and money spent on illnesses may be saved. What could it hurt to try it? I sometimes even dare people to drink distilled water for one week and promise to pay them back for the cost of the water if their sicknesses do not improve. I have never had to buy water, yet.

Now, to take it a step further, what type of water should you drink: distilled water, rainwater, spring water, or even tap water? People relate that they drink all kinds of water, and they have reasons for drinking it. However, I posit that human beings are organic creatures. Therefore, foodstuffs that go into the body for food or for liquid should also be organic.

What am I saying, the reader asks? Some types of water are "hazardous to health" (**Walker, 1974**). That is because the minerals that are found in spring water and mineral water are inorganic. These miniscule particles have been absorbed and dissolved into the water, but they are still in their whole parts, and once they come together with other granules just like themselves, they begin to form larger and larger pieces, until pebble-sized particles are developed. Eventually, the drinking water that is inorganic, whether mineral or spring, has all of these little, miniscule particles of calcium, iron, or whatever metal they may be - little rock-like, sand-like particles- that begin to accumulate where? In the kidney and in the gallbladder- and, eventually, a person has kidney stones and gallstones. Why: Because the body cannot break down these inorganic minerals.

On the other hand, however, the minerals that are to be broken down by the body should come through the soil into the vegetables and fruits, and the sun works upon them and turns inorganic matter into organic minerals and vitamins. Then, when people eat fruits and vegetables, that's how they get their minerals. Minerals and vitamins were not originally designed to be extracted from water. Water is meant to be drunk, so that it, in a clean and clear form, may enter the system to completely cleanse, revitalize, and give the cells their functions.

So, what kind of water should everyone drink? It should be distilled water. I will not write about the best kinds of distilled water – there are two that I talk about when I have personal consultations, but in this written format I will just say this: Each person needs to study his or her locale to find a distillery that is reputable to get the best distilled water possible. My research has convinced me that this statement is factually true: Distilled water is what a person should drink.

The next question might be this: Should cold or hot water be drunk? Remember, normal body temperature is 98.6 degrees, and, if hot water is being consumed as in hot tea, and it is being drunk quickly into the system, it can literally scald, burn or cause a catastrophic reaction. This may happen when a liquid that is well over 100 degrees enters a body which is only 98.6 degrees. Ingesting this heated substance forces the system to try to cool off, which may set the system up for some serious illnesses.

On the other hand, when ice cold water is drunk or ice is bitten into, there is a common reaction that feels as if an ice pick has been slammed into the body. That is graphically the truth. Why should one get so much pain from something that is supposedly so good for him? The reason the pain occurs is because the substance is too cold for the body. So, the liquids or foods that are consumed should be lukewarm to cool. How does a person get the water cool? The distilled water jug should be set on the floor because, in most homes or buildings, the floor is the coolest area in that building. If the water is set on the floor, it will be relatively cool. It should not be hot; it should not be ice cold. Which brings up this issue: making tea. To make tea, the water should be warmed just enough to not aggravate or cause a caustic reaction to the system.

I repeat this information over and over because it is most important that these points are remembered:

1. Room temperature water to cool water should be consumed.

2. People should not drink water that is composed of inorganic minerals, such as spring or tap water.

3. Distilled water should be the water of choice for consumption. If distilled water is impossible to acquire, the next water of choice should be purified water; and

4. A person should drink water that has been cleansed by reverse osmosis. If distilled water is unavailable or difficult to acquire.

5. One important point to remember is that when using filters to cleanse water it is next to impossible to know exactly when the filters are ineffectual. That is why distilled water is the best water to drink. However, in lieu of drinking no water at all, a person needs to just drink the water of choice. Yes, "bad" water is better than no water at all.

Now, what is the formula for the optimum daily amount of water each person should drink?

1. A person should take his body weight;

2. divide that in half; and

3. drink that number of ounces of water per day.

For example, a man who weighs two hundred pounds should drink 100 ounces per day. This is four more ounces than 12 glasses of water per day, or ideally about 12 and a half glasses of distilled water per day for his body weight. To concretize this formula, use this example: Taking a woman who weighs 130 lbs: Formula: 130 pounds divided by two equals 65 ounces of water per day. This approximates a half gallon of water per day, or 8 glasses of water, which is ideal for her body weight.

Finally, there are some who have stated that there are some doctors who advocate the mere drinking of liquids, i.e., tea, juice, milk, etc., as being acceptable for optimum health. During the health seminars that I conduct, I choose a person in the audience to tell me the name of his favorite drink. Afterwards, I ask the person to state the kind of car he drives. My point of not merely drinking liquids to wash one's body is further visualized when I ask the person this: Would he wash his car with that favorite beverage? This causes an eruption of laughter, but the bottom line is that most people treat the washing and caring of their cars as more important than the care of their bodies' internal organs. I know that, if that person were to find someone washing his car in the kind of liquid with which he washed his own body, he would fuss, cuss, and, possibly, kill because those liquids would, literally, wear the paint off the car. Still, everyone feels that it is fine to use juice and tea inside of their bodies as the major cleansing fluids, instead of pure, distilled water.

The body is made up of over 65 - 75% water. A person's bones are 30% water. One gets rid of a quart and a half of water per day in basic movement. How does that water get replaced unless a person drinks pure, distilled water? It is shameful to walk around with a dried-out interior. And still, most people wonder why they feel less than optimal most of the time. Many are almost a case of dry bones who need to 'hear/read the Word of the Lord.'

Finally, I will close this portion on the intake of plenty of water with a discussion of chronic fatigue, a prevalent problem with a lot of people. Signs of chronic fatigue include being tired all of the time; also, people find out they forget things and do not know why. I have a simple answer for the situation. People who suffer from chronic fatigue are not getting enough oxygen into their systems. That's the bottom line: There is not enough oxygen going to the brain and to the blood cells. That's where water could play a most important role, for water is H^2O; so, whenever you drink water, you are drinking millions of molecules of oxygen, sending them straight through the system, straight up and around into the bloodstream and straight to the brain where they belong.

Also, the use of water is excellent in the treatment of various headaches, muscle tension, and digestive complaints. Speaking of the latter, it would do a body good to sometimes just simply drink water for a meal. That's right, if a person's stomach is bothering him/her, and it is time for dinner, he/she might do well to say "no" to dinner, at that time, and "yes" to a nice, room temperature glass of water. If that same ill person could go and relax for about 30 minutes, he/she might feel better. I am speaking from what I have witnessed. Water helps with many digestive problems.

So, there it is: Water *washes*. Water *cleanses*. Water *rejuvenates*. Water *revitalizes*. Water is the drink from Heaven that is sure to assist the body in all of its necessary functions.

Chapter 3

Being Temperate

> *And every man that striveth for the mastery is temperate in all things. Now they do it to obtain a corruptible crown; but we an incorruptible.* **1 Corinthians 9:25**
> *And be not drunk with wine, wherein is excess; but be filled with the Spirit...* **Ephesians 5:18**

The well-known American writer, William Cullen Bryant, lived to a very old age. When asked the reason for his exact Health at such an advanced age, he replied, "It is all summed up in one word: moderation." **Paulien, 1997**

The third letter of the B.I.B.L.E.W.A.Y. acronym is another "**B**". This "B" stands for "being temperate". *Mirriam-Webster's Dictionary and Thesaurus* defines "temperance" as "a noun that means moderation/ abstinence or self-control in thought, action, or feelings". If any Christian was asked about the word, "moderation", he or she could possibly, easily spout off the words to the scripture about '*doing all things in moderation and nothing in excess*'. This has been the Christian rule for thousands of years. The Bible does not combine those thoughts together. Christians did that and it appears to be a pretty good rule. However, it is not. Read this with a prayerful spirit: if a person can do everything with moderation, and nothing in excess that means one can have a little nip of gin, from time to time; he can smoke a little bit of crack: people can even experience adultery every now and then, as long as they do not overdo it. Is the point being taken? If you can do all things in moderation, that's not good for a Christian. Paul was counseling to "be temperate" in all things. This means that we should shun that which is harmful. That is not like the scripture that speaks about being able to do all things through Christ. That use of the word "all" is good and healthy. Yes, one can even learn to do Christian things in moderation because that would be included in the all things that one should strive to do. Am I making any sense?

There's a scripture that says that *a little honey is good for the stomach's sake.* It says a little honey. So, if honey is good, and it is a fact that honey, as opposed to white sugar, is actually a food that is good for the body, to have to eat a little of it makes a tall statement. It is a sweetener of which God desires that His people partake. The Bible even talks about the Christians' future homeland flowing with milk and honey. The bottom line is that the scriptures refer to a little honey being good for thy stomach's sake. What is that saying? That's saying that, even if something is good for a person and ordained by God, He only wants that thing dealt with in moderation; He leaves no room for error. God does not ordain the excess use of anything.

Another meaning of temperance is restraint. A person should hold himself back from overdoing or excess. One should abstain from substances that are harmful. Sometimes self-monitoring would mean that a person might have to mentally pop his own hand, if he found it reaching for another piece of chocolate cake or a little red wine. Never mind that popular personalities suggest that a glass of red wine is just what's needed for women's health. What does God say about alcoholic beverages? They are definitely not to be consumed, to extinguish the risk of being one who is mocked. Abstinence saves lives.

How about those things that are not good for a person. If the things that are good are to be done in moderation, what is to be done about things that are not good for a person? Again, most Christians believe that as long as they do not overdo temptations, a little bit will not hurt. Let me use the bathtub as a first picture in this situation. Visualize a bathtub with its enamel finish actually eaten away by a constant drip of water in one spot – month after month drip-drop, drip-drop, year after year. Water dripping that way, one drop at a time, can actually eat a hole in a porcelain tub. If that is truly the case, then what will a little bit of sin do over a long period of time? Or, in this case, what will a little bit of wrong eating or wrong drinking do over a long period of time?

The principle is the same. Is it not known that over a period of time, doing something wrong, even in small amounts, will eventually add up to something catastrophic? That is how cancer and other diseases evolve. They begin with small things that are done wrong over long periods of time which weakens the body. Next, the life's forces begin to ebb away because the immune system just cannot handle it anymore. It cannot fight off the onslaught of effects materials, or poisons and toxins that have been built over long periods of time.

So, there it is in a nutshell. God wants His people to do things that are good for them in moderation. Things that are not good for them, they should not do them at all, contrary to popular belief. Period. That is the way of the Christian.

Further, the scriptures relate that the marriage bed is sanctified by God because its purpose is to bring forth children; it is what God gave to his beloved. Even sex, however, taken out of its spiritual context and even overdone in the marriage, can become a truly disastrous thing in a marriage. Many marriages have been destroyed when one partner took the sexual activity to an excessive state. This, again, shows that that which is good for a person, if overdone, is not good for anyone.

Again, I will reiterate that the Christian should do that which is good for them in moderation, and that which is not good should not be done at all. They should not eat too much; a person should not work too much; and one thing that destroys relationships is when another person talks too much. No, that should not be done. God gave mankind two ears and one mouth which means that God intended for people to listen twice as much as they talk.

So, if one thought is gleaned from this section on "be moderate" let it be that, if a food or an action is questionable, total avoidance is a rule of thumb. Why not err on the side of right?

Temperance means moderation or self-restraint in the indulgence of natural appetites and passions. We are told: "With our first parents, intemperate desire resulted in the loss of Eden. Temperance in all things has more to do with our restoration to Eden than men realize." **White, 1951**

Chapter 4

L ots of Rest

> *The sleep of a labouring man is sweet, whether he eat little or much: but the abundance of the rich will not suffer him to sleep.* **Ecclesiastes 5:12**

The work of building up the body takes place during the hours of rest. In fact, one might say that the biggest part in the recovery of disease is the rest the individual gets while recuperating. Rest invigorates and renews. Tired nerves need rest... **White, 1948**

Lots of rest and sleep is what the "**L**" stands for in the acronym, B.I.B.L.E.W.A.Y. Ecclesiastes 5:12 states: *that the sleep of a laboring man is sweet, whether he eats little or much: but the abundance of the rich will not suffer him to sleep.* This shows that God gives his honest, diligent children, not just sleep, but sweet sleep. So, why is sleep so important, and what are the best hours of sleep? Why? To answer the latter question first, it is scientifically proven that when a person gets one hour of sleep before midnight that this one hour of sleep is equal to two hours after midnight. That's right. Then, there's Genesis 1:16 which reads: "And God made two great lights: the greater light to rule the day and the lesser light to rule the night: [H]e made the stars also". Now, what does ruling the night mean? Since the moon is the lesser light, how can it rule one's life by night? Let me remind everyone that I am not speaking of horoscopes or the stars and the moon and those created things being above God; I'm speaking of God's Word. It says that this lesser light would rule by night. How does that happen?

Well, it has been proven that the moon's gravitational pull on one's body between the hours of 9 p.m. and 3 a.m. is the greatest. That's when the pull is the greatest. This gravitational pull has been proven to put man into a deep sleep or R.E.M. sleep or rapid eye movement sleep. It's been proven that all of the hours of sleep before midnight are the best; the first three hours after midnight are the best hours of rest. Therefore, the best hours of sleep are from 9 p.m. until 3 a.m.

Many people say that they work the "graveyard shift", and, thus, are in a state of confusion about what to do. In that case, one would do well to get into bed early. Four or five hours of sleep before midnight or before his shift starts would leave him well rested. If it was possible to find another hour during the day to sleep, that would even out his lack of acquiring the best hours of sleep. He would be as well rested as possible.

What other conditions assist to produce a good sound sleep, thus helping the body function optimally?

Remember that good, sound sleep helps the body repair while a person is asleep. The nerves are strengthened; food finishes its digestion; the blood cleanses; and the kidney and the liver do their jobs of getting the poisons and toxins out of the body. They actually work harder while sleep is going on than when one is awake. The scriptures state that "the life of the flesh is in the blood" (**Leviticus 17:11**), and it takes blood for all of these bodily functions to work. So, when a person is asleep, his body gets busy. Again, all of the organs get busy cleaning, restoring, repairing, strengthening, and revitalizing the body.

Now, what types of things can a person do to produce this good sound sleep that will give him all of those benefits that were mentioned above? First of all, one should sleep in a cool room. If there's a choice between a hot, a warm or a cool room, always choose the cool room. A look at past experiences would probably reveal that all of the best sleep states a person has had were when the environment was cool or cold. In the wintertime, it's so cool sometimes that a person does not want to even wake up to go to the bathroom because such a sound type of sleep is being enjoyed.

Secondly, should the room in which one is to sleep be dark or well-lit? The room should be dark because it is proven that the body rests and the mind gets better sleep when a person is sleeps in a dark room. So, the television has got to be turned off. A person will never get the best sleep with the television on.

Thirdly, the choice needs to be made between a quiet room and a noisy room. Of course, one sleeps better in a quiet room. It's an absolute necessity. To go to sleep with earphones in one's ear to study or listen to the radio is not good because the mind is attempting to deal with the words and phrases that it is hearing, and the body is trying to go to sleep. This takes the body through a tug-of-war. The blood is trying to let the person rest so that it can do its repair work, and then on the other hand, it is trying to keep the person semi-awake so it can deal with the information that is going through the mind. This is a double taxation on the body. The room, therefore, that one sleeps in should be a quiet room.

Lastly, the room in which a person sleeps should have fresh air coming into it; so, if there is a window or two in the house that can be cracked so that good, fresh, night air can be coming in to move out the stale air and keep fresh air circulating into the room and into the lungs, this is a plus. It really is a must in order to get the best, good, sound sleep possible.

What happens when the room is just right for sleeping? One gets good, solid rest for his nerves. They rest in an undisturbed fashion, and the person awakes, not only physically ready to go, but mentally and spiritually ready to move the next morning because the nerves have rested undisturbed.

Besides a cool, dark, quiet room that is inundated with fresh air, the next thing to remember about invoking the best sleep is this: One should go to sleep on an empty stomach. There should be no food in the stomach four to five hours before one goes to sleep. Why? The digestive and eliminative systems are the largest ones in the body, starting at one's mouth and ending at the anus. It takes blood for them to work. If the body is going to digest food, it takes a lot of blood to do it. Has anyone ever noticed that, many times after a meal, people will get sleepy? Well, blood is drained from the head, and it goes to the digestive system to begin the digestion of food. So, if a person is trying to sleep, and the body is trying to digest food, there is not enough blood flowing to the brain to give a person an equilibrium that gives good sleep. Instead, the brain is starved for oxygen and blood, and the sleep is a most aggravated, agitated type of sleep; it's an unrestful situation.

Under the best conditions, which were just discussed, it has been found that an individual only needs four to six hours of sleep. Of course, babies and small children need much more because they are so active during the day. For the average adult, however, four to six hours would be great sleep under the best conditions. Eight hours is the average amount, however.

In closing, I'd like to point out that, just as the first three letters of The B.I.B.L.E.W.A.Y. acronym are definitely commands or prescriptions from God, so it is with this one, "Lots of Rest." In order to show that, I will go to the Bible where there are numerous instructions and prescriptions for "rest". One of the most significant ones is found in Genesis 2:2-3, which reads thusly: "After God had created the world in six days, He rested on the seventh day from all of His labor and all of His works that He had made." I fail to believe that He did this because He was tired. No, it was in order to show His people a pattern. He was showing everyone that He knew we would need rest from our labor; so, He rested from his labor, and He designated one day of rest at least one day out of the week when man could break away from the humdrum and from the rat race. That's right. He gave us an opportunity to rest from the 24/7 that we normally get into. Of course, this biblical subject of rest is highly controversial; therefore, we won't dwell too long on the ramifications it holds. Let every person be persuaded in his/her own mind, as he/she 'rightly divides the word of Truth."

It has been found, scientifically, that the body needs rest; it needs relaxation; it needs revitalization from the energy that is exhausted in the workplace. So, if rest is needed, and, if rest is not gotten any other way, God gave His people a day of rest. This is absolutely important. This needs to be, prayerfully, seen and realized that God would not have given His people that day, if it had not been important for them. Also, in Scripture it is found that God says in Mark 2:27 that the Sabbath was made for man, and not man for the Sabbath. So, here, God made this day for man to take a rest. There is nowhere in the Bible that says, as many people say: "When Jesus died, he nailed the Sabbath commandment to the cross"; or "that day is not important, because it was for the Jews"; or "God does not mind a person choosing his own day on which to rest... "

Even, scientifically, it has been proven that when a person works six days and rests the seventh day, he can work the other six days with a lot of vitality. People who work seven days a week, however, have been found to have much shorter life spans, and are more prone to sickness and disease.

So, all of the points in the chapter "Lots of Rest and Sleep" are to be taken seriously. Please, also, everybody consider the need to do as God did and commanded that His people do: one day out of the seven-day week span, set aside a day for rest from labor. No, not to worship the day, but to be obedient and follow Christ's undeniable example.

Rest strengthens labor and labor sweetens rest. **Wilson & Wilson, 2010**

Proper periods of rest are part of an intelligent system of treating disease. **White, 1948**

Chapter 5

Exercise Daily

And the Lord God took the man and put him into the garden of Eden to dress it and to keep it. **Genesis 2:15**

You'd have to go a long way to find something as good as exercise as a fountain of youth. And you don't have to run marathons to reap the benefits. Little more than rapid walking for 30 minutes at a time, three to four times a week can provide ten years of rejuvenation. **Harrell, 1991**

The next prescription for health is represented in the B.I.B.L.E.W.A.Y. acronym by the letter "**E**", and it is found in Genesis 2:15: *"and the Lord God took the man and put him into the Garden of Eden to dress it and to keep it."* So, it is observed that, in the beginning, after God had made the perfect man, a perfect being, created in His own image, one of the very first things that He did was to place the man in the Garden of Eden to tend it. How did he do that? Basically, he kept the grounds of the garden; he was a gardener who kept the, possible, leaves swept up; he picked up fruit that may have fallen to the ground. I submit that the first man was a farmer, because God knew that, even though this body was perfect, even though it was designed to live forever in the beginning, it still needed exercise to keep it a perpetual machine. That new body was like a brand-new automobile: it would have become inoperable, if it just stayed parked in the driveway for a year without even being turned on. However, with a little running, even as minute as backing it out and taking it for a short run up the street and back, that car, more than likely, would crank after the year was up. Activity was needed for that automobile. Likewise, activity also keeps the human body working in an optimal condition.

For the average person who is in reasonably good condition, exercising twenty minutes a day is sufficient to maintain physical fitness. A body's basal metabolic rate slows down from two to three percent every decade after age nineteen. It is said that a low metabolic rate tends to increase lifespan, and, with moderate exercise, a person can achieve the maximum oxygen volume of a person fifteen years younger. With a higher degree of regular exercise, the oxygen volume of a person forty years younger can be achieved. Those people who exercise feel better about themselves than those who do not. It improves their self-image, as well as their mental sharpness.

"Since exercise is such a wonderful thing for our bodies and such a necessity, let's talk about the best form of exercise. One of the simplest, natural, inexpensive, controlled, and strengthless exercises is walking. We are

told that there is no exercise that can take the place of walking. By it the circulation of the blood is greatly improved." **Paulien, 1997**

"When weather permits, all who can possibly do so are to walk in the open air every day, summer and winter. Walking, in all cases where it is possible, is the best remedy for diseased bodies because in this exercise, all of the organs of the body are brought into use." **White, 1938**

Walking stimulates thoughts by increasing the brain's supply of oxygen, and it lifts or elevates one's spirit through the release of natural mood elevating chemicals called endorphins. Walking, I say, is, therefore, better than medicine, for it is known that *"a walk even in winter would be more beneficial to health than all of the medicine the doctor may prescribe"* (**White, 1938**). This quote falls right in line with the fact that walking as a prescription helps to control weight and makes one feel much better. The plus is that there are no ill side effects under normal conditions.

Walking is also a natural body healer, as discussed in the following excerpt: "Walking acts as a natural bronchodilator, releases chest congestion, helps the body expel toxic wastes and improves breathing capacity. If a person experiences shortness of breath, this is nature's indication that his body needs more oxygen. A greater need for oxygen is found; by slowing the breathing down and concentrating on exhaling, one may restore oxygen to her system more rapidly" (**Paulien, 1997**).

Increased oxygen that comes from walking is absolutely essential to restore vitality in the body and to natural body healing. How much walking is necessary, and how fast should one walk? The goal for a person to be able to walk at a good brisk pace for about twenty minutes. His cardiovascular level should be up to approach almost being out of breath, i.e., not being able, hardly, to hold a conversation. When a person gets to where he can do that, he is in good shape; he's at a point where the body can really utilize the intake of oxygen, and the benefits are going to be that he will have greater mental capacities and be physically stronger with more stamina.

The following quote is proof that walking is everybody's opportunity.

"Walking is the tranquilizer without a pill. It is the cosmetic not sold in a drugstore. It is therapy without a psychoanalyst. It is the fountain of youth that can extend {one's} lifespan. It is the vacation that doesn't cost a cent. It is the exercise that needs no gym. It is the gym that needs no equipment. It requires no lessons from the pros. It requires no expenditures beyond the price of an extra pair of shoes a year. It can take away anger and anxiety, solve a problem and untangle physical and psychological knots. It can be engaged in individually or in groups. Its time is anytime. Its place is any place. And it fits into anybody's and everybody's schedule."

"Such exercise would in many cases be better for health than medicine. Physicians often advise their patients to take an ocean voyage, to go to some

mineral spring or to visit different places for a change of climate, when in most cases, if they eat temperately and take cheerful, healthful exercise, they would recover health, and would save time and money" **(White, 1951).**

Chapter 6

Wonderful Sunshine

And God made two great lights; the greater light to rule the day, and the lesser light to rule the night: he made the stars also. *Genesis 1:16*

Sunshine is death to all disease producing agencies, and it is life and health to all natural forms of life. **Paulien, 1997**

Since Christ is also the physical and spiritual healer, he is called the sun of righteousness. *Malachi 4:2*

The "**W**" in the acronym by the way, is all about 'Wonderful Sunshine'. God placed His *greater light in the sky*, according to Genesis 1:16, *to rule the day*. That light, the sun, has various purposes, the most important of which is to give light and warm the earth for the continuum of life.

Sunlight seems to be the mother of all of nature's processes. God made the sun to be the source of all energy in this world, which makes it necessary to all physical life, growth and healing. The following are some of the sun's effects on our bodies' life functions:

1. Sunlight lowers excessively high blood sugars, which gives the pancreas a rest and increases proper and complete digestion of food.

2. Sunlight lowers blood pressure and increases circulation by bringing more blood to the circulatory system. This means less work for the heart and more rest for the heart between beats, thereby lowering the risk of heart failure. Also, the resting heart rate will decrease and cause the heart rate to return to normal

much more quickly after exercise. When this happens, there's a decrease in lactic acid in the bloodstream, which reduces soreness in the muscles.

3. Sunlight also changes cholesterol beneath the skin into vitamin D, where it is stored in the liver until the body needs it. This does two things. First, it decreases blood cholesterol levels; this, in turn, reduces the future possibility of strokes and arteriosclerosis, and for bypass operations. Secondly, Vitamin D helps with the body's absorption of calcium, a nutrient which strengthens the bones, nails, teeth, and skin.

4. Sunlight also reduces arthritis symptoms by loosening the joints.

5. Although exposure to sunlight increases the skin's ability to resist diseases such as acne and psoriasis, one must be sure to avoid free fats and hydrogenated oils, margarines, and shortenings, which minimizes the possibility of acquiring skin cancer.

6. Exposure to sunlight boosts the immune system by creating more white blood cells and stimulates the liver to detoxify poisons in the body.

7. Sunlight causes wounds to heal faster and better by keeping them germ-free; and

8. Walking or bathing in sunlight helps to eliminate disease-causing agents such as cancer and AIDS by increasing the ability of the blood to absorb oxygen. Diseases fail to thrive in a medium of oxygen. I will expound on the knowledge that oxygen has a destructive power over disease in the next chapter.

It has been found that many beneficial effects of sunlight are heightened, if a person practices a regular program of physical exercise and combines it with sunbathing. Reportedly, blood output is increased by an average of 39 percent for several days after sunbathing. Of course, too much sunshine is detrimental, too. I advocate that spending a minimum of fifteen minutes in the sunshine - allowing it to shine directly on the face and the hands – is a sure way of obtaining an adequate amount of sunshine for the sake of health.

Sunlight is a desired weather state more so than dark clouds. That is shown by the fact that people seem to move more spontaneously and easily on sunshiny days. Not only is temperament improved through sunlight, but an added plus may be that the body's immune system is strengthened by sunlight. However, if for no other reason than that it is just plain good for the bones, habitual obtaining of sunlight is a bonus to sound health practices.

In closing, based on the above conclusive list of the benefits of sunlight, this scripture deepens in meaning: **Malachi 4:2** states, *But unto you that fear my name shall the Sun of righteousness arise with healing in his wings; and ye shall go forth, and grow up as calves of the stall.*

Chapter 7

Air, Fresh and Clean

> *And the Lord God formed man of the dust of the ground and breathed into his nostrils the breath of life; and man became a living soul.* **Genesis 2:7**

Fresh air will prove far more essential to sick persons than medicine, and is far more essential to them than their food. They will do better and will recover sooner, when deprived of food than when deprived of fresh air. **White, 1938**

The letter *A* is always in the beginning. So, it is with the letter *"A"* in the acronym *B.I.B.L.E.W.A.Y.*

When man was first created, the first thing God did was: ". . . *breathed into his nostrils the breath of life; and man became a living soul*" (**Genesis 2:7**). Without his breath, man is dead. Air is just that important. To attempt to live without it would be foolishly impossible.

Since the air is so important, why is it taken for granted? Yes, air's importance is taken for granted: It is filled with pollution on a continuous basis - so much so that the government has to admonish businesses and corporations to adhere to strict clean air practices. There is only one environment to last a lifetime on this earth; so, man needs to see that it is kept as clean as possible.

What is the best air to breathe in for the sake of health? Good air is electrified. That's right. The life-giving oxygen molecule is negatively charged or "ionized". There are many remarkable effects to living in an environment of negatively charged ions. These include improved functioning of the lung and its protective cilia; lower resting heart rate; improved learning in human beings and other mammals; decreased anxiety; decreased survival of viruses and bacteria in the air; and decreased severity of stomach ulcers.

The above listing lets me know that everyone needs as much fresh air as possible. Case in scenario: When life begins to get the best of a person, he could feel a lift in his spirit by getting out of the city and finding a nice spot in which to just go and breathe in and breathe out - i.e., at the park or at the seashore (or lake shore). Ideally, owning a home in the country would likely benefit an entire family, also.

Furthermore, people should learn a technique of breathing that contributes to optimal body maintenance and function. Which brings up this next topic: oxygen cocktails. I coined that term as I taught audiences the following variations of a simple, well known breathing technique. Breathe in very slowly through the nostrils while counting to four. Hold the breath for two seconds and exhale very quicky while counting to four. Since this pattern promotes clear thinking and calm nerves. I had an epiphany moment that automatically pronounced that this way of breathing should be called an oxygen cocktail. Procedurally, more oxygen is being forced into the diaphragm; the shoulders stand more erect; the posture is, therefore, better, and more oxygen is going to the brain. Many body parts work more effectively because of this breathing technique that gets more oxygen into the body.

This is a personal testimony: Our special needs child was often plagued with lung problems and congestion problems until we found a spacious home in the country. In that atmosphere of clean, "negatively charged", fresh air, Jesse Hezekiah thrived as never before. During a checkup following our move, the nurse listened to his chest and back, checkpoint after checkpoint, and was shocked that he sounded so 'clear'. Is not God the God of fresh air, also? Going outside to breathe will work wonders for your health – especially in the fresh morning air.

Chapter 8

Y ield to God's Will
Always

Trust in the LORD with all thine heart; and lean not unto thine own understanding. In all thy ways acknowledge him, and he shall direct thy paths. **Proverbs 3:5-6**

"All who consecrate body, soul, and spirit to God's service will be constantly receiving a new endowment of physical, mental and spiritual power. The exhaustible supplies of Heaven are at their command. Christ gives them the breath of his own Spirit, the life of his own life. The Holy Spirit puts forth its highest energies to work in heart and mind." **White, 1948**

The *"Y"* in the acronym, *B.I.B.L.E. W.A.Y.*, represents *"Yield to God's Will Always"*. How appropriate it is to end this acronym with one of the last letters of the alphabet – if all of the other prescriptions are accepted and followed, and this last prescription is neglected, a person has just 'spun his wheels in neutral'. His health will always be in jeopardy because he is not a committed Christian. Without Christ's life as mankind's object lesson – or his pattern – he will never be whole. His body may be the healthiest, but his spirit will lack vitality and luster.

Biblically, there are many examples of how the heeding and yielding to God's will is the safest place for Christians. If God says, "Go"; one had better go! If God says, "Stay", a person would do best to stay! If God says, "Wash", washing would be in order! If God says, "Stand", to not stand would not be an option!

Who would be a better example than Naaman, the captain of the host of the king of Syria (**2 Kings 5:1**). Naaman was a mighty man of authority and valor, who probably commanded the respect of all of Syria, being the captain of the king's army. He had to come down from his high-status pole, however, when he met Elisha, the "prophet in Israel". God's prophet advised him of the only way he would be cured of the deadly disease, leprosy, which is centered around the Y in B.I.B.L.E. W.A.Y. Naaman had to YIELD to God's will.

In synopsis, Elisha tells Naaman to *go and wash in Jordan seven times, and thy flesh shall come again to thee, and thou shalt be clean* (**2 Kings 5:10**). Because the Jordan was not composed of quality water, Naaman, initially, refused to go and *dip in the water*. As a matter of fact, Naaman became quite angry! After his own servants pointed out his foolishness in not following the simple prescription of *washing to be clean* in the Jordan. Naaman *went down and dipped himself seven times in Jordan, according to the saying of the man of God: and his flesh came again like unto the flesh of a little child, AND HE WAS CLEAN* (**2 Kings 5:14**).

Most times, God does not require a person to perform some long-drawn-out deed in order to outwardly show that he will follow God's will. Many times, people with less education or social status will be able to follow God's will before those of the upper echelon. Why? That is just the trickery of the devil to fool them into believing that they are able to be gods. Really. It may be that some of those people believe that they "pulled themselves up by their own bootstraps"; therefore, they may not feel a need to depend on or rely on or trust in God. "I did my way" is a stand that many worldly people acclaim. Who made the sun that is shining on them? Who made the water that they drink? Who made the air that they breathe?

Yield: To submit; to surrender. On one hand, it seems that yielding would be hard to do. On the other hand, to be able to yield gives the connotation of ultimate freedom. Concerning the former, one who is full of pride finds it hard to admit to needing someone else's help. Do I have examples of any cases, where people who are full of pride would rather drag around in sickness than to admit being vulnerable to needing God? Yes, I do. Other examples have presented themselves where an ill person just could not stand the thought of receiving directions from the Lord from me. I only shake the dust off of my feet from such negative spirits and allow the Lord to use me in the health of those who *will* accept me as God's health evangelist.

Whether therefore ye eat, or drink, or whatsoever ye do, do all to the glory of God. **1 Corinthians 10:31**

The previous point about yielding is shown vividly in the demeanor of a wild horse and the procedures used in training him. Visualize a horse that is bucking, kicking, and frantically attempting to throw the rider each time he attempts to ride him. This happens for a period of time. Then, one day, the horse appears to submit instantaneously. He had been ridden so much in his wild state that he seems to gladly become rideable. He yields to the rider. He appears to be at peace from struggling. He accepts that he is a horse who has been caught (called) to a life of service and obedience. So, it is with man toward God. It requires the cessation of struggling against God to yield to His will. God, too, is happy that the man is ready to listen to His commands and directions – freely. The fight is over.

Unlike the horse trainer, God does not force his will upon man. Man decides for himself – through choice – that God is the rightful Force to which to yield. Man realizes that he cannot live a life of freedom without God's protective hand covering him. Knowing that God will allow no ill to overtake man that will not be for his "good", man is able to ride through evil and all of the wickedness in high places that will attempt to conquer him. Man, further realizes that fighting against God is utter foolishness, and that attempting to exist without Him might end in man's destruction.

The Bible is chock-full of numerous examples of people who found peace and victory after yielding to God's will. From Genesis to Revelation, reading all the stories of patriarchs and prophets, kings and commoners, and disciples and followers gives current believers a hope of glory. That belief filters over into the health realm, also. Since I started on this journey of health for

God, I have come to accept that, as with Naaman, many people find it hard to just do the simple prescriptions that God outlines for them to achieve health: All any person has to do first is to surrender and yield to God's will – always.

The basis of *The B.I.B.L.E.W.A.Y. to Health: Prescriptions from the Great Physician*, promotes simple remedies for optimum health.

B - Best Foods and Combinations

I - Intake of Plenty of Water

B - Be Temperate

L - Lots of Rest and Sleep

E - Exercise

W - Wonderful Sunshine

A - Air; Fresh and Clean

Y - Yield to God's Will Always

It does not always require running through hoops or jumping over boulders; God has a will for each person's life, and, as the saying goes, "He knows how much a person can bear". He does know. Many believe that God will not allow a health problem to overtake a person for which there is not a way to escape or overcome it. Timing is very important, but trust is the main ingredient needed in yielding to God's will. If one would really believe that God is a God of mercy and grace, and that He desires all to 'be in health and prosper', that person would also be extremely attentive to the timeliness required in overcoming many ailments. Once a person realizes that, many times, overcoming a sickness naturally requires a strict   regimen a minimum of three months, he needs to access a plan immediately.   For instance, cancer is a sickness that develops over time: Just as the sickness developed over time, it may take a while to be "cancer free".   Does that make common sense?

Although I do not make a big splash about it, I am one of God's vessels of aid to sick folks. There are certain herbal remedies and formulas that I have been blessed to put together – that through documented cases - work.

Most are just as simple as opening the kitchen cabinet and refrigerator to pull out lemons and garlic and other such healing kinds of foodstuffs. They are all considered the "right stuff" for wellness.

I yielded to God's will for my life over forty years ago. I will not say that God's will has been appetizing all of the time, but I will say that yielding to God's will is best and safe. I have also accepted that being a medical missionary is not the most lucrative calling in life, but my family has never been hungry, nor has anyone of my family been naked. "God is good all of the time; all the time, God is good." His will is the best. He loves all of humanity equally and waits for all to hear the gospel message – including the health message - so that He may claim and/or reclaim those who want to be with Him.

Bleak pictures are painted of those who will not yield to God's will concerning the health message. One such picture includes the woeful look of a person riddled with cancer, who could not/would not overcome an addiction to cigarettes. He was "a sucker" for cigarettes.

The air that he breathed in with each suck was almost like a brick being laid to construct the foundation for a body riddled with cancer. Realistically, such a person would need to be committed to a natural plan of healing for a longer while than a person who was following a plan to be healed from the flu.

It's amazing, also, that many foods that people consume are on God's forbidden list, i.e., in Leviticus 11, there is an outline of all flesh meats that man was commanded not to eat. God told man to not even touch the pig: Instead, what does man do? He eats the pig from his snout to his feet, and he uses parts of his body for aids, i.e., boar bristle brushes. This transgression has meant a death sentence for many people. Picture this: With each chew of pork meat, man might swallow numerous worm larvae that travel throughout the body, connecting to various organs, i.e., the lining of the colon to, eventually, cause all kinds of medical problems. I understand that many autopsies expose the sewer-like conditions of a body riddled with worms and larvae. And many people are expecting to offer that up to God. He said do not eat or even touch the animal. Man eats it, touches it, and expects God to accept it. That is food for thought.

Answer this, though: If your child consistently and constantly disobeyed you, would you accept that behavior? I could go on and on painting various ghastly pictures that show how the body responds to blatant disregard for God's prescriptions for health . . . Can the reader relate to this statement: Love is responsible for a lot of ill health? I know that I have yielded to the will of my children every now and then – and I allow certain food items to be consumed, knowing that they were not the best choices, many times resulting in later dental issues that needed painful rectification. When I do that, I am no better than anyone else. Just as the reader loves his children, God loves the reader. He allows His children to have the "freedom of choice". So, no, I cannot point a finger at the reader because 'there, but for the grace of God, go I'.

I will stop at the above view – without expounding on the person in the picture who could not put literal fat meat down, and who, therefore, is blind and crippled - attempting to exist, as digit after digit and toe after toe, even foot after foot is chopped off (or amputated, to make it more palatable) – due to diabetes.

I will not tell you that the bent over man in the corner of the picture refused to drink his water or eat to his calcium-rich foods as a young man - claiming that calcium was for sissies – and this is his lot to walk in a constant bow to God – possibly to make him, now, mindful that God is to be reckoned with sooner or later. Oh Yes! The day of reckoning will come for every man, woman, boy and girl. Prayerfully, everyone will be able to stand when the time comes.

Will it not be pitiful to have this commentary to make: "I read Dr. Franco's book, but I was not ready to accept his suggestions. After all he is just a man as I am – or so I thought. I am in this terrible shape, physically, all because I would not eat the best food and combinations; I refused to drink water or practice moderation in my lifestyle; I had too much to do to get adequate rest and sleep; exercise was not on my agenda – light or strenuous; I ran from the sunshine, and for me to take a minute to breathe in the outside air was unheard of. All of this amounts to the fact that I did not/would not yield to God's will – not even for a day, not to mention for always. Then in the end I cry out to the Lord, "Please take me to heaven with you just the same!"

The sad part is going to be that sin is sin. To reject the light of scriptures concerning physical health is as serious as the rejection of the light of spiritual health. Hopefully, your mind will turn to God in health matters. High blood pressure does not have to be hereditary – that yoke of bondage can be broken – as proven time after time. AIDS does not have to become full-blown just because a person has been pronounced to have the HIV virus. A child with cerebral palsy does not have to live under the bondage of lung and mucus problems. I am speaking what I know from experience or what I have seen – not only from what I have heard.

Everybody, come on and YIELD TO GOD ALWAYS. Health is yours, for the asking.

There is only one sure remedy for the transgressions of life, and that is to be brought face-to-face with the fact that mankind has a Maker who designed each type of cell in the body, planned their functions, arranged their nutrition, gave and continues to give that mysterious thing we call life and some every day will call every person to account for the treatment meted to the "image" of his Maker. The acceptance of this truth gives vitality to the conscience which calls man to loyalty to his Maker. **White, 1951**

Bibliography

Batmanghelidj, F. (1997). *Your body's many cries for water*. Vienna, VA: Global Health Solutions, Inc.

Bragg, P. C. & Bragg, P. (1970). *The shocking truth about water*. Burbank: Health Science.

Buettner, D. (2008). *The blue zones*. Washington, D.C. : National Geographic Society.

Diehl, H. & Ludington, A. (2011). *Health power: Healthy by choice, not by chance!* Hagerstown, MD: Review and Herald Publishing Association.

Gibbs, G. (1993). *The food that would last forever*. Honesdale, PA. Paragon Press.

Goodness Lover, LLC. (2021). *The gut/brain solution: episode transcripts.*

Harrell, C. C. (1991*). In search of the fountain of youth.* Memphis, TN: Health Forum Publishing Company.

Jackson, T. A. (2024). Menopause: My story, your journey—A practical solution on how to address menopause the natural way.

Jensen, B. (2000). *Guide to diet and detoxification.* Lincolnwood, IL: Keats Publishing.

Kloss, K. (2005). *Back to Eden.* Twin Lakes, WI: Lotus Press.

Nedley, N. (M.D). (1999). *Proof of positive: how to reliably combat diseases to achieve optimal health through nutrition and lifestyle,* Ardmore, OK.

Paulien, G. B., (Ph.D.). (1997). *The divine prescription and science of health and healing.* Brushton, New York: TEACH Services Inc.

Reader's Digest. (1997). Foods that harm, foods that heal: An A-Z guide to safe and healthy eating. Reader's Digest Association.

Merriam-Webster. (2023). Merriam-Webster dictionary
and thesaurus. Merriam-Webster, Inc.

The Thompson chain reference bible. (5*th Ed.)* (1988). IN:
B.B. Kirkbride Bible Co.

White, E. G. (1931). *The place of herbs in rational therapy.*
Message Press, Coalmont, TN.

White, E. G. (1941). *Christ's object lessons.* Review and
Herald Publishing Association Takoma Park:
Washington DC.

White, E.G. (1938). *Counsels on diet and foods.* Takoma
Park, Washington, DC: Review and Herald Publishing
Association.

White, E.G. (1951). *Ministry of healing.* Mountain View,
CA: Pacific Press Publishing Association.

White, E.G. (2003) *Medical ministry. (*2nd ed*).* Mountain
View, CA: Pacific Press Publishing Association.

White, E.G. (1948). *Testimonies for the church*, Volumes 1-9, Pacific Press Publishing Association.

White, J. G. (1951). Abundant health. Northwestern Publishing Association, Sacramento, CA.

Wilson, M. & Wilson, D. (2010). *Back to Adam.* Savannah, TN. Centurion Ministries: Savannah, TN.

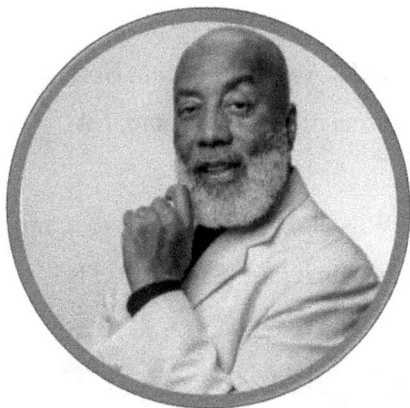

Bro. Dr. Franco Taylor

Bro. Dr. Franco Taylor, I.H.E.*, is a servant, like his Elder Brother, the Lord Jesus Christ, and, in 1980, was called to be an *international health evangelist or medical missionary in this world where rising medical care costs and escalating pharmaceutical costs are forcing people to seek answers for their health problems through alternative methods of healing. He is on call 24-7, six days a week.

Who is he?

He is a counselor who ministers to the whole person: spiritually, intellectually, physically, and mentally. He is a teacher who advocates his own brand, "the B.I.B.L.E.W.A.Y. to Health", teaching biblical ways to be well and stay well. Bro. Dr. Franco is a nurturing father to eight grown children (one is deceased, Frank Christopher), four of which he delivered at home; and he is the loving husband of one wife, Linda.

Who is he?

Bro. Dr. Franco is a God-fearing, Bible-believing Christian man who realizes that his people are perishing because many are unaware that the Scriptures hold the keys to health and happiness. He realizes that all men are created equally, and has found that all men, equally, have to accept that sickness knows no color - diabetes, high blood pressure, heart disease, obesity, cancer, etc., attack the just and the unjust. This noted businessman, master baker and vegetarian food designer has produced an all-natural food and supplement line through his family-owned business, Right Stuff Health Ministries, Inc.

Pedagogically, he attended the public-school systems of Chicago, Illinois and Memphis, Tennessee. After graduating from Central High School in Memphis, he studied pre-med at Maryville College in Maryville, Tennessee. Later, Bro. Dr. Franco acquired practical health care experience by working as an aide at several health sanatoriums (the last of which was the Centurion Bible School of Health, in Cypress Inn, Tennessee, operated by his mentor and confidante, Bro. Mamon Wilson). Later, from 2006 to 2016, he acquired a Bachelor of Holistic Health and Nutrition (B.H.H.N.) from the Indian Board of Alternative Medicine (IBAM), a Master's degree in Herbalism (M.H.) from the, then, Clayton College of Natural Medicine in Alabama, and the coveted Naturopathic Doctor degree (N.D.) from IBAM. In 2021, he received certification as a health practitioner from the American Naturopathic Medical Certification Board.

In 2017, he was nominated and selected to receive the President's Lifetime Achievement Award, signed by President Barack Obama.

In culmination, Bro. Dr. Franco has delivered the good news of the health message by conducting seminars and health "revivals" for individuals, businesses and churches in the United States and abroad. Through this act of evangelism, many souls have been saved as they come to believe that, as stated in 3 John 2: 'God wishes above all things that His people be in health and prosper, even as their souls prosper'.

For information concerning individual consultations, seminars or revivals contact us at 901-383-0404 or info@rightstuffhealth.org or www.rightstuffhealth.org

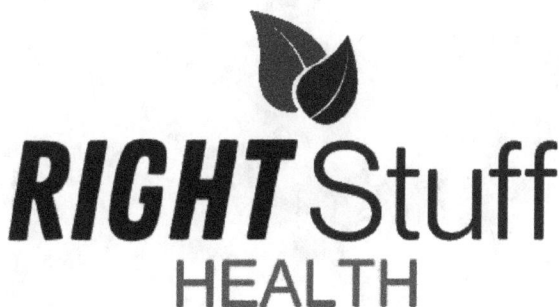

RIGHTStuff
HEALTH